DR ELEWECHI

How
I Stood Up
To
CANCER

Empowering Women to Overcome Life's Challenges

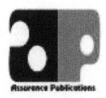

Assurance Publications

Published by Assurance Publications Ltd,
P.O. Box 112, Washington, NE37 1YB
United Kingdom

Tel: 07799653641

Email: info@assurancepublications.com
http://www.assurancepublications.com

Available from Amazon.com, Amazon.co.uk and other retail outlets

FOREWORD

The dreaded "C word", the "big C"; these are some of the ways we start our discussion when it relates to cancer. It is truly a dreadful disease but should we always cower to it? Can we stand up to it? Yes, we can. This is what Dr Ngozi Okike is telling us in this book. She uses her faith in God together with the medical expertise that is available to her to 'stand up' to this dreaded disease.

I have been in medical practice for over 20 years as a Breast and General surgeon. Over the years I have noticed that patients who show an 'inner strength' either through faith or self-determination always do well. To have this clearly expressed by a patient, will be an encouragement to all past, present and future patients.

One of the things that I like in the book is how Ngozi carefully described and explained in a 'layman's language' the intricate processes that the medical personnel have to go through in reaching a diagnosis and formulating a management plan. This shows the excellent practice that the British National Health Service (NHS) offers. She also subtly points out some aspect where hospitals could do better and perhaps anybody reading this book, who happens to be admitted to hospital should take this into consideration – noisy wards.

There are many different types of cancer and different causes. Some are genetic or hereditary, some due to environmental causes and in most cases an interplay between the two. The precise nature of this interplay or interaction is not known in the medical field. What is known is that we can positively shift the outcome in our favour by keeping to a healthy lifestyle in what we do and eat. Dr Okike gave a good measure of this advice in her book.

Although Dr Okike has used her personal challenge, breast cancer, as a basis for this book, the principles expressed in it are applicable to any type of disease, whether malignant (cancer) or not. In fact, they are applicable to any challenges we are facing in life.

iii

Whether you are a person of faith or not, and it does not matter the faith, whether you have been treated or are receiving treatment for any form of cancer or going through any form of challenges in your life currently or you just want something to encourage and uplift your spirit, this book is for you.

Folajogun M Oluwajana MBBS, FRCS
SAS Breast and General Surgeon
Chesterfield Royal Hospital
Chesterfield, UK.

Preface

We live in a world full of uncertainties. Many of those who have read my book *'The Greatest Debtor to His Love and a Trophy of His Grace,'* no doubt arrived at the same conclusion as the BBC Tyne Reporter, Sarah Hathaway, who described my life as 'dramatic and eventful.' She made this remark after she visited our home a second time for a video interview with me. She confessed that she found some of my life's stories rather fascinating, and that if she could, she would come to our home again and again to do video interviews with me[1]. Indeed, the story of my life from my mother's womb has been quite dramatic. I count myself rather fortunate to still be alive in spite of some of the dramatic events I have encountered, many of which still make me shudder when I remember them. I recall a few people who, when they were reading my book, commented that the book had 'gripped' them. My neighbour said he felt like coming to knock on my door to ask what I had done to his wife; he could not get her attention anymore, as she was literally glued to my book. It is a blessing that many have found courage and strength from the pages of this book.

I hope that much more than *'The Greatest Debtor,'* readers of this new book, *'How I Stood Up to Cancer'* will find it even more inspiring. The title of the book itself tells the story. Usually when someone is told that they have cancer, their whole world falls apart; everything changes, and a big battle begins. How this battle is won depends on the state of our minds and the words we speak to ourselves. How do you react to such news? How do you prepare yourself for the journey into the unknown that you're about to embark upon?

---

[1] See
http://www.bbc.co.uk/tyne/content/articles/2007/09/28/tyne_abortio n_video_feature.shtml, and
http://www.bbc.co.uk/tyne/content/articles/2007/04/19/video_natio n_escapefromslavery_video_feature.shtml.

My 'journey' began when I woke up on the morning of Tuesday, October 9, 2012 and felt a lump on my right breast. Following this discovery, I was about to embark on the toughest journey of my life, so far. As you read this book, I pray that it encourages you to not give up despite what you are facing, and gives you the strength to believe that things can get better. As more and more of this drama unfolded, I knew it was for a purpose, and that I would have to write about my experience at some point. Interestingly, most people really close to me suggested that my experience could really help many others in a similar situation. Many of them said to me 'don't worry; another book will come out of this experience.' The story of how I missed the opportunity to be one of the Torch Bearers during the London 2012 Olympics is published in my book, '*The Torch Bearer: Two Sides of the Story*;' In '*The Torch Bearer*', I talked about how we can inspire others in spite of the challenges we face in life (including dealing with cancer), like one carrying a bright torch in a dark room.

In this book, '*How I Stood Up to Cancer*' I share how I won the battle with cancer - in my mind, and in the words I spoke to myself. I hope that many who read this book will find strength and inspiration to know that even if you are unfortunate enough to be diagnosed with cancer, your life still has purpose and meaning. You too can stand up to cancer and move forward with your life by having a positive mental attitude and saying the right words to yourself. How is that possible? I encourage you to read my story. My prayer is that as you walk through my journey, you will be inspired to face your situation with a winning attitude.

I must admit that describing some of my experiences in this book has been an emotional rollercoaster. A few times I have found myself in tears all over again, as I have tried to recall some of the challenges I faced. My only consolation is that many who will read this book will find it to be truly inspirational and appreciate what it is to be confronted with a diagnosis of a rare type of cancer, especially when it arrives so unexpectedly! More importantly, I hope that all who read this book will understand what it is to 'stand up to cancer' by not allowing it to get the better of you. Like every other battle, cancer can also be won with the right mental attitude, the right words and a good diet. No one goes to battle with defeat on the agenda. In a similar vein, you can win your battle with cancer – in your mind.

Elewechi Ngozi M. Okike

ABOUT THE BOOK …

This is a truly unique and moving book. It is one that takes the reader through a private and daunting journey, which many take but almost always remains unspoken.

One enduring message which is summed up in this book, that even recent advances in medical sciences is not privy to is the power of the human spirit, and how it relates to events of our life particularly in the outcome of difficult events.

Time and time again the author stresses that she would not let her condition disrupt her life adversely or stop her life from normal activity. Her working right through the entire radiotherapy treatment and also having minimal reaction from the therapy evidences this. A general observation I made for quite some time now as someone who sees hundreds annually is that often you can tell those who will do well by their courage and fearless spirit. As a result, this book has ministered to me personally and also I am certain there is something unique there for all who read it.

Mr Obi Iwuchukwu, FRCS FRCS (Gen) MD
Consultant Breast & Oncoplastic Surgeon, Sunderland Royal Hospital, UK

****

Breast cancer is a devastating diagnosis to give a patient as a doctor. It is life changing when it affects you personally, causing you to reflect on many things, including family life, personal goals and your own mortality.

As a consultant physician and a husband, whose wife received a breast cancer diagnosis, Dr. Okike's book is very resonant in my own life.

She is honest and open about her emotions and her struggle to find God's way forward in the storm. Her story will inspire and inform you. She gives insights into the process you may go through, as well as some important spiritual and health advice.

On a personal level, I can recommend Dr. Okike as a woman of God who lives as she writes - full of passion and determined to help others along the journey.

Dr. Andrew Davies (consultant physician) MB BS FRCPE

****

This is indeed a fascinating read, really arresting and life inspiring.

Dr Goke Aiyegbayo, MD Rickleton Medical Centre, Washington, UK

****

A diagnosis of breast cancer is devastating for any one. In this book Dr Elewechi Okike describes how her close family network and strong faith helped to equip her with the strength to be able to work through her individual breast cancer journey and beyond and is now able to share her experience within this book with the aim of helping others in the future. As her Macmillan Breast Care Nurse I was in a privileged position to help support her throughout this challenging time.

Michelle Derbyshire
Macmillan Breast care Nurse

****

From a pathologist's point of view making the diagnosis of this unusual type of breast cancer was a challenge.

The book is a heart-warming read for everyone, giving the reader a close perspective of someone suffering from cancer and a real feel how the strength of human spirit and character can help to beat the disease.

Dr Mona Jain, MD(path), MRCPath
Consultant Histopathologist.

****

It is with great pleasure I recommend another book from Ngozi Okike. Her life story is always full of surprises and the Lord has used her testimonies to inspire many to overcome where they would have succumbed. Jesus changes lives and this book will inspire you to trust him in the face of cancer. The world needs to hear that cancer bows before the name of Jesus. Read on!

Pastor (Dr) Timothy Dunnett
Senior Pastor Bethshan Church

****

Ngozi Okike is truly a woman of faith. In this book she tells of her battle against rare cancer and how she triumphed. For those needing courage and inspiration, this book is a must read.

Pastor Ken Gott
Senior Apostle Bethshan Church

****

I am absolutely elated to endorse Dr. Elewechi Okike's latest book; *"How I stood up to Cancer"*.

As I began to read through the chapters, I was so captivated by this personal real life challenging experience that I could not stop reading until I read the whole book in one sitting. Never have I encountered such a woman who time and time again has exemplified what it truly means to live and exhibit a life of total faith in the true and Living God. It is one thing to be suddenly diagnosed with such a horrendous disease as Cancer but to also be told that it's one of a rare kind is yet another blow to any human mind. Yet she faced this giant with courage, bravery and a strong leaning on God.

There are many who have faced this challenge of similar or even less magnitude and unfortunately did not live to testify about their comeback from the disease. I am sincerely grateful to God for this amazing overcomer. However, as a result of her standing up to this giant, she not only conquered but is now living to tell about the journey and how others can be victorious too.

Three distinct outlooks I discovered through out her incredible journey is her ability to embrace the challenge with such positive attitude, absolute faith and trust in God to get her through this, and her declaration. She consciously made a decision that this diagnosis was not going to get the best of her. She then embarked on relying on God's promises and standing firmly with confidence on God's Word. Lastly, she chose to declare what God's positive word said and not the negative report.

I admire not only the careful narration of details of her journey, but also in each chapter she brought hope and assurance that it does not matter how grievous and bad the situation is, you can overcome it. Dr. Okike's tremendous strength and tenacity to face this giant head on and win goes to show why she is so passionate about helping others by sharing her story.

The most intriguing chapter amongst many others was chapter 4: "Life at the ward". She was in the valley of the shadow of death, none could go with her except the One who never leaves us and never forsakes us. This was a defining moment for her, life could go one way or the other, but she stood firm and at that very moment God gave her "Life at the Word". His Word sustained her. While reading this particular chapter which also brought me to tears, I was reminded of a very powerful scripture found in Proverbs 4:22, "*for they are life to those who find them and health to one's whole body*". It describes how we are to pay attention to the Word of God, embrace it and tuck His Word in our hearts. His Word brings health to our whole body.

Isn't it just like God to not only take you through a gruesome ordeal but He always brings you out greater than when you went in, hence taking this victory all the way to the British Medical Journal. It is now written, recorded and firmly established that what a loving and caring God did in Dr. Okike's life, can never be forgotten for years to come and lives will be changed as a result; bringing glory to God.

I commend Dr. Okike for her heartfelt story of how she defeated a giant called Cancer that stood in the way to disrupt her destiny. I have no doubt that the lives of anyone who picks up this book will be changed forever. It's remarkable; it's encouraging, and totally life-changing.

Dr. Chidi M. Kalu

President
Light Strategic Coaching
Windermere, Florida

Dedication

This book is dedicated to all those men and women who helped and supported me during what would appear to be one of the darkest periods of my life. It is also dedicated to all those who are being treated for any form of cancer, and to those whose lives will be touched and transformed through reading this book.

ACKNOWLEDGEMENTS

Although I did not share my experience with cancer with many people, a few of those who got to know about it did their best to help. Appropriately therefore, I would like to use this opportunity to express my gratitude to all those who stood by me and supported me and my family in so many ways, either through visits, phone calls, the provision of food and much more with their prayers, during what has been one of the most difficult and challenging periods in my life. These include Drs Onyebuchi and Pat Eseonu, Dr Myra Herbert, Dr John and Mrs Margaret Ameobi, Chief Sonny and Mrs Suzanne Iroche, Drs James and Betty Nwabineli, Dr Olamide Olukoga, Mr and Mrs Mode, Mr Jonas and Mrs Comfort Abladey, Margaret John, Mr Charles Uwakaneme, Professor Nsidinanya Okike, Mr Ogbonanya and Rosemary Okike, Mr Steve and Mrs Vera Ailemen, Ms Temitope Fodunrin, Pastor and Mrs Bolaji Ismail, Dr Francis and Amaka Ndaji, Dr Chidi Kalu, Mr Kalu Omokwe, Mr Cyril Asuquo, Mrs Christy Omoruan and many more too numerous to mention. Drs Onyebuchi and Pat Eseonu deserve special mention for the role they played in my life, and the support they gave to me and to my family; and the sacrifice they made financial and otherwise. May the Lord you have all honoured in the sacrifices that you made and the love that you showed, reward you mightily.

Special thanks also go to my GP, Dr Goke Aiyegbayo, The Consultant Oncoplastic Surgeon, Mr Obi Iwuchukwu, the Macmillan nurse, Michelle Derbyshire and all the other doctors, nurses and radiographers who took care of me. It is because of the role they played that I have a story to tell. They ensured that I received the best possible treatment, care and attention. I am indeed grateful for all their love, care and support.

I would also like to express my appreciation to our son, Helmut Okike, for his insight and for giving the book the professional touch it required. Our daughter, Adaeze, did a lot of work in editing and proofreading the contents of this book. I'm grateful for her input.

Words are inadequate to express my gratitude to Dr Folajogun Oluwajana, for his contribution. In spite of his very busy work schedule, he found the time to read through the drafts of this book a few times to ensure the accuracy of the medical narrative in the book. I am indebted to him.

Finally, I want to thank my immediate family for the role they have played in my life and for all the love, understanding and support they gave to me during this difficult time. My husband and children rose to the challenge, and were there for me any time.

Most importantly, I'm grateful to God, my Father, for His very special grace in my life that enabled me to stand and face the cancer challenge head-on. I could not have done it in my own strength. All the glory goes to Him alone.

CONTENTS

LIST OF ABBREVIATIONS

Bible Versions
NKJV – New King James Version
NIV – New International Version
ISV – International Standard Version
ESV – English Standard Version
CEV – Contemporary English Version
NLT – New Living Translation

(Note: All translations are from the NKJV of the Bible, unless otherwise specified).

SRH – Sunderland Royal Hospital
MDT – Multi-disciplinary Team

Chapter One

An Unforgettable Day

There are certain events that occur in our lives that are unforgettable. The discovery that I made on the 9th of October 2012 opened up another chapter in my life. I recall that the BBC Reporter, Sarah Hathaway, had described my life as 'dramatic and eventful' following a couple of interviews she did regarding the story of my birth and my escape from abduction during the Nigerian Civil War. However, even after all I have encountered in my life, little did I realise that another major drama was about to unfold.

Many of us who travel regularly by plane often do not pay attention to flight attendants when they go through their usual safety drills informing passengers about what to do in an emergency. This is because we have heard it so many times, we feel it is a routine exercise and never really expect to be in a situation where we may be required to recall this information.

Recently when I heard about a plane that had landed on water, I tried to imagine how the passengers may have reacted. They would have been required to implement the safety instructions, which they may have previously ignored. Similarly, this is what happens when we attend talks or seminars that teach about caring for our bodies, and carrying out routine health checks. Often we don't take these teachings seriously until we are faced with reality.

I recall attending a women's conference in 2009 in which we were reminded about the need to examine our breasts regularly, and taught how to do so. Now and then I did try to carry out this check, but I did not do this regularly. However, I recall lying in bed on the morning of Tuesday, 9 October 2012, feeling an urge to examine my breasts. I examined the left one and it appeared to be fine. However, when I examined the right one, I had a very strange feeling. A sudden panic came over me as I tried to figure out whether what I was feeling was real or imaginary. What does a lump in your breast feel like? I was not very sure.

My regular GP was male, and therefore to be thoroughly sure, I thought that the female nurse in his surgery might be in a better position to tell me whether what I felt on my breast was a real lump or something else. When I tried to make an appointment at my GP's surgery to see the nurse, I was told she had no free slots until Friday, 12th October. I was very uncomfortable about waiting until Friday for this strange thing in my body to be checked. When I told the receptionist at the surgery that I needed to see the nurse urgently, she then enquired as to why I needed to see the nurse. I explained that I had felt a lump in my breast and that I needed to have it examined to be certain of what it was. The receptionist advised that I would need to see the GP, not the nurse. Unfortunately, I could not see the GP earlier than Friday, so I accepted the first available GP appointment which was on Friday, 12th October at 3.10pm.

It is impossible for me to quantify the emotions I felt as I thought about the potential diagnosis. I knew that quite a few women die from breast cancer, including some personally known to me. Up until this time, I had never heard of any member of my immediate or extended family that had suffered from breast cancer. So, where did this strange lump come from, and why me? These thoughts were going through my mind. What if the doctor said it was a real lump? Would it be life threatening? I knew this was going to be a real battle, if it turned out to be so. Was I mentally, emotionally and physically prepared for what this was going to demand of me? As a Christian, I receive strength from my faith, so after spending some time in prayer, I went about my business as usual, looking forward to the appointment with my GP to try and unravel the 'mystery.' Apart from my husband and children, I am not sure I mentioned it to anyone else.

On Friday 12th October, I went to see my GP as scheduled. He was a Christian and someone well known to the family. The

Practice Manager was also present in the room when he examined me. He looked at me with mixed emotions and a deep sense of compassion and told me that it was a real lump. In other words, this was not my imagination; it was real! Of course I was speechless. I felt tears falling down my cheeks. He gave me some tissues to stem my tears and said that he prayed all would be well, and explained that there was a possibility for the lump to be benign. He then asked me to go and see the Practice Nurse who would try to secure an appointment for me to see the Consultant at Sunderland Royal Hospital (SRH) within two weeks.

The Practice Nurse was very sympathetic, as she had been in the same situation about sixteen years ago. Fortunately the lump in her breast was benign and she had not experienced any problems since then. She also tried to encourage me, saying she hoped it would be benign, and that there would be nothing to worry about.

I got an appointment to see the Consultant on Monday, 22nd October. When I got home I told my husband all that had transpired. We prayed and committed the whole situation to God. Until proper tests were carried out there was nothing to worry about, as we had no idea whether or not the lump was benign or malignant. As far as I was concerned, life continued as normal. However, deep down I couldn't believe that such a thing was happening to me in the first place.

I'm aware that many do not believe in God or the existence of darkness or evil. As a Christian, I believe in God, and I know that sometimes certain events happen which cannot be explained. I was determined not to allow this situation to have the better of me and believed that God would see me through this situation.

Interestingly, my husband and I travelled to London shortly after seeing my GP that day. We had an engagement in London that weekend, as our friends were having a 3-in-1 celebration, including a big party for the husband who had been cleared of pancreatic cancer. Yet here I was waiting to find out the nature of the lump in my breast. Nevertheless, the news we heard did not detract nor dampen our spirits. The trip would go on, as planned. As a matter of fact, we stopped off at Luton, en route to London, and visited some family friends. We also visited two other families in London that weekend. No one knew I was facing a personal challenge, as I appeared upbeat and well. I was as happy and cheerful as always, just as though nothing was happening with me. We had a wonderful time in London, with gratitude to God that we were able to make the journey.

Besides the trip to London, we were also planning a very important event, one which dignitaries from across the country were being invited. The 5th Anniversary celebration of Book Aid for Africa (BAFA), a charity which I founded in 2007, was coming up on the 27th of October, less than three weeks after I had found a lump in my breast, the nature of which was still being investigated. We held regular BAFA meetings, which I chaired. This was a very busy time in my life, and in spite of what was happening to me personally, my cheerful demeanor was not dampened. Although I chaired most of the meetings, there was nothing in my disposition to suggest that I was going through a personal challenge. We never know what people around us may be going through so we must never judge or jump into conclusions just based on eternal appearance, which highlights the importance of giving people the benefit of the doubt.

I had been referred to a Breast and Oncoplastic Consultant, and given an appointment for the 22nd of October at Sunderland Royal Hospital. Tests were required to ascertain whether the lump I had found was benign or malignant. It was an anxious time. Nevertheless, I went about my business as normal. I have always felt so secure in the love and the kindness of God, and I knew that He was with me on this journey.

Chapter Two

The 'Journey' Begins

When I received my appointment letter to see a Consultant at the Sunderland Royal Hospital on the 22nd of October, I was delighted to find out that I had been referred to a Consultant I already knew. That was reassuring. Interestingly, I had gone to work as usual, and my husband came to accompany me to the hospital. We met with the Consultant Oncoplastic Surgeon, who examined me and asked me to do a mammogram, scan, and other tests. During this first visit, a triple assessment was done. First was the examination by the Consultant, the diagnostic mammogram and then an ultrasound scan. This diagnostic mammogram is different from the screening mammogram that women undergo as part of the preventive measures against cancer. It focuses more on one area of the breast, providing views from several angles at higher magnification. It also helps to investigate the lump and other symptoms, such as any tissue thickening, skin dimpling or nipple inversion. The Consultant needed this mammogram done to pinpoint the location and size of the lump in my breast.

Having identified the location and size of the lump as seen on the mammogram, I had to have an ultrasound-guided biopsy. The ultrasound creates images of the inside of the breast on a monitor, and helps to determine whether the lump in the breast is fluid or solid. The Consultant said the biopsy was necessary to ascertain the type of lump found in my right breast.

However, as I lay down on the couch during my biopsy, and watched the radiographer conduct the test, I could not but wonder at what was going on in my body as the picture I saw on the monitor was rather bizarre and inexplicable. In carrying out the biopsy, the radiographer used a special needle to draw a sample of tissue from the suspicious area of the lump in my breast. After the biopsy, the tissue taken from the suspicious area of the breast is sent to the lab for analysis. It could be cancerous, a benign or non-cancerous lump, or the nature of the lump may not be clear. In my case, the tissue drawn from the lump in my breast was slimy, with the appearance of liquid glue.

I did all the necessary tests and was asked to return two days later for the result.

When we returned on 24th October, I was pleasantly surprised to be informed that the lump appeared to not be cancerous. Of course we were very delighted at the news. That is the kind of news most people pray to receive in this situation. He also added that the Consultant Histopathologist who carried out the test on the specimen of the lump had said the type of substance found in my breast was rare, and that she had never seen such before. Hence the Consultant indicated that the removal of the lump needed to be performed urgently so that further tests could be carried out to determine the nature of the substance within the tumour. I was then scheduled for surgery on the 6th of November.

My right breast was still feeling sore as the biopsy was carried out under local anesthesia. Whilst this 'drama' was unfolding in my life, the 5th anniversary celebration of BAFA was scheduled to take place on the 27th of October. I carried on with my life as normal – intertwining hospital visits with making plans for the anniversary celebration. Thankfully, the event was successful; no one knew the personal challenge I was facing. A battle was going on in my life, and being won in my mind, which no one knew about. My faith in God continued to help me to stand strong.

I had important appointments in the south of the country during the first week of November. I was meeting with the High Commissioner for Mozambique in London on the 2nd of November to discuss how BAFA could support underprivileged schools in Mozambique. In addition, my role as a PhD External Examiner required me to examine a PhD thesis in Bournemouth on the 5th of November. Yet, I was scheduled for surgery on the 6th of November? How would that be possible? I was concerned that I would not be mentally, physically, or emotionally prepared for surgery after such a hectic few days. I needed to mentally prepare for the challenge ahead. More importantly, I needed time to pray! I knew there was no way I could go for surgery on the 6th of November. I rang the hospital just before I travelled to London to let them know I would need to reschedule the operation on the 6th of November. The Personal Assistant to the Consultant was surprised because she knew the Consultant was keen for me to have the lump removed sooner rather than later.

After I got back from my trip I knew I needed some time for prayer, self-reflection and self-examination. It was important for me to express how I was feeling in prayer and obtain strength from God.

Like most women, I always went for my regular breast screening. The last one I had in March 2011 confirmed that '*your mammogram appeared normal in that no signs of breast cancer were seen. This means that your next routine screening appointment will be due in three years' time.*' Unfortunately, less than 18 months after this report, I found a lump in my breast, which could be cancerous. What could have happened between the last mammogram and the most recent one?

My mother, grandmother, great-grandmother and other females down my family line never had breast cancer. Where on earth did this come from? I needed to gain some spiritual insight into what was going on in my life; I needed to find an answer from the Bible about my situation. I gained strength from a few bible passages: John 11:4, '*this illness isn't meant to end in death. It's for God's glory, so that the Son of God may be glorified through it* ' (ISV); Luke 21:13, '*This will be your opportunity to bear witness*' for me (ESV). Wow! I felt really encouraged. In addition, I read and memorised another bible reading from the book of Psalm 118. Some verses of that chapter were very reassuring

'*And so my life is safe,*
  and I will live to tell

23

what the Lord has done
(Psalm 118: 17 CEV).

Having been so reassured, I felt rejuvenated and full of faith that this situation would end well.

Besides spending some time in prayer, I took the Holy Communion EVERY DAY. For Christians, the Holy Communion symbolises the death of Jesus Christ. In the Bible it states in Isaiah 53: 4-5 '*He suffered and endured great pain for us, but we thought His suffering was punishment from God. He was wounded and crushed because of our sins; by taking our punishment, He made us completely well*' (CEV). So, when we take the Holy Communion, we are affirming our faith in Him, and claiming all the benefits and promises, including good health; the assurance of peace in the midst of life's challenges, and many more. Therefore, by taking the Holy Communion everyday, I was reminding myself of this fact, and appropriating the benefits.

Prior to all these developments, Psalm 91 in the Bible was a Psalm I prayed DAILY. I was particularly encouraged by verse 10 which says '*no evil shall befall you, nor shall any plague come near your dwelling,*' Verse 15 of the same Psalm says '*he shall call upon Me, and I will answer him; I will be with him in trouble; I will deliver him and honor him*'? I believe God hears when I pray and I know His love for me is total and complete. Whatever was going on in my life was only a temporary challenge.

Again, for Christians, we see the Bible as a 'lamp unto our feet, and a light to lighten our path.' I received a lot of strength from the Bible during this difficult time, and found the passages I read to be full of hope. One of the stories that encouraged me as I was reflecting on my personal challenge was the story of Job. In the Bible, Job was described as '*a truly good person, who respected God and refused to do evil.* (Job 1:1, CEV). Yet, he went through a lot of hardship and difficulty at one point in his life, however he trusted God, and everything that was taken from him was completely restored. He received so much more than he had lost.

24

Interestingly, prior to the discovery of this lump, I had been nominated to be one of the Olympic Torch Bearers for the London 2012 Olympics, but other commitments did not permit me. However, as the games drew closer, it dawned on me that I had missed a once in a lifetime opportunity to carry the very famous and prestigious Olympic Torch. Little did I know that I was being appointed as a 'Torch Bearer,' from a completely different perspective, one that carries the light of hope?

The Consultant was not happy that I was unable to attend my surgery on the 6th of November. We met with him again on the 9th of November and he still insisted that I needed to have the surgery. I struggled with the thought of undergoing surgery. Why could I not believe that God could heal me and I would not have to endure an operation? Could I not believe that God could make the lump disappear? Interestingly too, the Consultant himself was a Christian, just like my GP. I felt this was a blessing from God.

I believe in healing, and I believe in miracles. I have prayed for people and they have been healed. There have been many times that I prayed for myself and been healed, so why could I not believe that God could remove the lump? These were the thoughts going through my mind. I decided to go ahead with the surgery and trusted God's involvement in the whole process.

After we met the Consultant on the 9th of November, he arranged for me to have the lump removed on the 20th of November. He was scheduled to go on a two-week holiday, and wanted to perform the surgery before his holiday. Therefore the surgery was booked for 20th November. However, between the 9th and 20th of November, there were quite a few social events and activities I needed to attend, and yet there was no indication that I was going through this challenge. Most people that I met or spoke to had no idea that I was facing a life-threatening illness. For me it was important that the small group of people that knew about my situation, were full of positivity and hope. I write later in this book about the power of words and the mind.

Before I went for the surgery on the 20th of November, I mentioned it to my Line Manager. Fortunately, he did not ask me for more details, but it was important that he knew I would be away from work for a few days. The Consultant had mentioned that many women reacted differently to the treatment. Some returned to work immediately, whilst others stayed home for a few days. I was not sure what would happen in my own case.

I attended church on Sunday, 18th of November, following which I informed the leader that I was going in for surgery on Tuesday, and he prayed with me and my husband. I also mentioned it to another couple in the church, but told no one else. My husband accompanied me to the hospital on the day of the operation. It was day surgery, and I was home later in the evening.

Chapter Three

'Are You on Your Own'?

After my excisional surgery (that is, after the lump in my breast was removed) on the 20th of November, I returned to Sunderland Royal Hospital (SRH) on the 28th of November for my post-op review, and to have part of my stitches removed. The SRH Histopathologist advised that she had never seen the type of lump removed from my breast before! I wasn't quite sure how to receive this news. The multi-disciplinary team (MDT) had met and was discussing the best way forward with my case. I did wonder why a multi-disciplinary team was needed.

Usually people with breast cancer are cared for by a team of professionals who bring their expertise into the care of the patient. The team includes:

- A breast care nurse, who is trained to provide information and support to anyone diagnosed with breast cancer;
- A surgeon (who carries out the surgery;
- A radiologist (responsible for the x-rays and scans);
- A pathologist (who examines the tissue and cells removed during a biopsy or surgery);
- A medical oncologist, who specialises in treating cancer with drugs;
- A clinical oncologist, who specialises in treating cancer with radiotherapy and drugs;
- A chemotherapy nurse, trained to give chemotherapy drugs;
- A therapeutic radiographer (trained to give radiotherapy treatment); and
- A research nurse, who can discuss the option of taking part in clinical trials.

Depending on the type, and the stage, of the breast cancer, the MDT can also include:

- A plastic surgeon;
- An oncoplastic surgeon (who is a specialist in plastic surgery);
- A physiotherapist;
- A prosthesis fitter (who helps to fit an artificial breast following a mastectomy); and
- A pharmacist.

In the mean time, due to the rarity of the type of lump in my breast, they decided to send the specimen to the Regional Consultant Histopathologist at the Queen Elizabeth Hospital in Gateshead. I was a little bit surprised, and kept wondering what was unfolding. Imagine how you would feel if you were in my shoes and heard that your case required regional attention. I kept reminding myself that God was with me, and I was not facing this ordeal alone.

The Consultant surgeon had mentioned that he would be away on holiday the following week, but I had actually forgotten this when I returned to SRH for my next appointment on the 6th of December. This time I met a different doctor who was with a Macmillan nurse. It just so happened that in addition to sending the specimen from my lump to the Regional Histopathologist, they had also sent it to the National Histopatologist!! Now, this did really shock me, and I knew that this was not an ordinary case. However, due to work commitments, my husband could not accompany me on this visit, so I went on my own. The doctor asked me if there was anyone with me, I replied 'no,' but in my heart I knew I was not on my own, and believed that God was with me. He then told me they were still awaiting the result from the National Pathologist, but the Regional Pathologist had said the test results showed a rare form of depressed cancer. Wow!!! This was the news I was dreading!

Although there are more than 200 types of cancer, breast cancer is the second most common cause of death from cancer in women in the UK. Nearly 12,000 people die from breast cancer in the UK every year, according to the Charity, Breast Cancer Care. How would you feel if after you had been told that the lump found in your breast was benign, to now discover it was cancerous, plus an extremely rare form of cancer? This was why the doctor had asked if I was on my own. He was going to give me the type of news that would require someone to be there with me. I took a deep breath and whispered a prayer. I felt a lump in my throat. I wanted to cry but did not know how. I was lost for words. The doctor left the room, and I was with the Macmillan nurse. You could see compassion written all over her face. Indeed, she understood what it is like to receive such news. That is the purpose of her training, to look after people who receive such news and to be there for them. I was now embarking on a journey that nothing had prepared me for. (Now I'm really trying to hold back my tears as I write this, as the memory is too painful). Despite the news, I was determined to remain positive, and believe that God would turn this situation around. There have been many instances where I have felt God's protection over me, and this time would be no different.

My case was unique; as a result the MDT was discussing the way forward, and how best to provide the right care for me. The interesting thing of course was that in spite of my surgery, and the uncertainty about the nature of the cancer I had been diagnosed with, I was back to work as normal, even before I went for this appointment. The only thing I could not do was drive because of the pain on my right breast. However, on this occasion I drove to the hospital myself. People at work had no clue what was happening with me. They saw me come in and out of work as I always did, and I carried on with my duties as normal.

Now alone with the Macmillan nurse, she asked about the general state of my health, my age etc. When I told her my age she said I did not look my age at all, for which I thanked her.

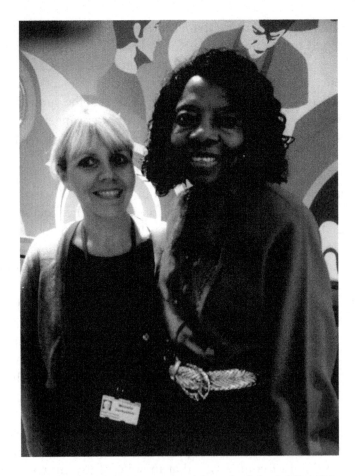

Elewechi and Michelle Derbyshire, the MacMillan Nurse

The nurse told me that I would have to undergo some blood tests and would need to come back the following week for a CT scan. She said she would love to bring me in much earlier, if possible. She handed me her complimentary card, as well as a pack containing information about the treatment of breast cancer. I gave her my mobile number in case she needed to contact me to rearrange any of my appointments. She removed the rest of my stitches that day, and then I went on to have my blood samples taken. However, before she left, I told the nurse that I would be ok, and had faith in God to preserve me.

Interestingly, in spite of the news I had received, and the numerous tests I had to do, I returned to the University and resumed work as normal. I was determined that cancer would not control my life.

The next day, surprisingly, I received a strange text message from one of the young ladies I mentor. She was asking about my general welfare because she had a dream about me, in which I appeared seriously ill. I encouraged her that when she has such dreams she should pray and ask God to keep that person safe, so that the dream does not become a reality. However, deep down, I was quite taken aback by this dream, but not surprised because I believe that sometimes God gives people dreams about a certain situation to encourage them, that He knows about their situation, and is with them. Given the enormity of the situation with my health, I decided to spend most of that day in prayer, and also took the Holy Communion.

My husband and I were back at the radiology department of the hospital on the 11th of December for my CT scan. This was a staging CT, to be sure the breast tumour had not spread to any other organ in the body and that there was no other organ from which the tumour could have originated. This was necessary, because of the rare nature of the lump in my breast; the diagnosis was in question. We went back the next day to see the Consultant Oncoplastic surgeon for the results of the tests as well as to find out if they had heard from the National Histopathologist.

I was still in disbelief that my sample had been required to be sent to the national Histopathologist! The Histopathologists at Sunderland Royal Hospital and the Queen Elizabeth Hospital, Gateshead, had examined the sample taken from the lump found in my breast and both of them had indicated they had never seen that type of cancer before. This was why the sample had been sent to the National Histopathologist. This time the wait for the results was rather long, and I was apprehensive.

The multi-disciplinary team meeting to discuss the type of treatment I would require went on for much longer than normal (over one and half hours). As we sat in the waiting area, I was wondering if the discussion was about me, or whether other cases were also being considered?

When we eventually met with the Surgeon that day, he told us that they had received a response from the National Histopathologist, who confirmed that the substance they found in the lump in my breast was rare, with only four such cases having been recorded in medical literature!! I was speechless, and prayed that this meant it would still be curable. He said the MDT decided that a wider local excision around the area of the breast which had been opened up would be necessary, and that he would also remove one of the nodes in my armpit. This was to take place on Saturday, 15th of December at 8.00am. I was asked to go and do a sentinel node biopsy the next day.

What is wide local excision (WLE)? When one is diagnosed with breast cancer, surgery is usually the first treatment to try to get rid of the cancer. The type of surgery will depend on the nature and stage of the cancer. The surgery can be either breast conserving, or mastectomy. With breast conserving surgery, or wide local excision, the cancer is removed together with some normal looking tissue surrounding it. In early breast cancer, having WLE followed by radiotherapy is as effective as mastectomy. However, if the cancer is at an advanced stage, a mastectomy is often recommended, followed by radiotherapy and/or chemotherapy, to ensure the cancer does not return. With mastectomy, the entire breast is removed and some or all of the lymph nodes.

Wait a minute! What does it mean to have a rare form of cancer, and why me? Although receiving this news was a shock, I knew that with the various situations I had encountered in my lifetime e.g., surviving abortion, escaping abduction, attempted murder etc. (all of which are detailed in my book *The Greatest Debtor to His Love and a Trophy of His Grace)*, I was not surprised that my diagnosis was rather unique; little did I know that more drama

32

would be unfolding. I had made medical history in the womb of my mother when I survived abortion, now it seemed I was making more medical history! I didn't know whether to laugh or cry.

Surprisingly, a few weeks after this appointment with the Surgeon, I received a letter from one of the surgical trainees at SRH who was part of the Breast Surgery team. He said that he was writing to me about my recent breast surgery because 'the nature of the lump that was removed is very rare' and that he would like my permission 'to write up the case for submission to a medical journal for publication,' He enclosed a copy of the proposed report, including some pictures of the lump. This request was rather surprising, and I did wonder what was going on, however I gave him the permission to do so. I felt that if my situation could help someone else, then so be it.

In everyday parlance, we all know what it is like, to 'open up old wounds.' These are certain issues or areas in our lives which are like 'tipping points.' They are sore areas, representing past events or happenings that we want to remain forgotten. I have a few of those myself, like my experience in Exeter in 1995, when I came face to face with man's inhumanity to man (again, full details in *The Greatest Debtor*). For some people it might be mentioning an ex-wife, ex-husband, or the loss of a loved one. Nobody likes to have old wounds opened up. So, when the surgeon told me he would have to go back to the spot where I had my first surgery and open it up again, I thought, 'this guy must be joking,' How on earth is that going to happen? I did not want to begin to imagine the pain that would be involved in this procedure! I knew I was in for something really serious, and the prospect of that surgery was very daunting. When we got home that evening, my husband rang up another doctor friend of ours, and he came to the house to see us. We told him what was happening, and he tried to explain why these additional measures were being taken. It was an extreme measure to ensure there would be no re-occurrence of the lump.

Chapter Four

Life at the Ward

I was back at the radiology department of SRH on the 14th of December and had a radioisotope injected by the nurse. This radioisotope injection would help the doctor identify the sentinel node to be operated on. This whole experience was opening my eyes to the fascinating world of medical science, and enabled me to see how much it has advanced.

December 15th was a day I had been dreading. Nevertheless, I chose not to be ruffled by this challenge I was facing, knowing that I was secure in the love of God, and that He had everything under control. My life was in His hands. Although the surgery on the 20th of November was a day case, this second operation was to take place in ward D47. I did mention to my Line Manager that I was going in for further surgery, and was delighted that he did not ask for details. So, again, I was saved from having to disclose that I was undergoing treatment for breast cancer. The point is that I did not like to talk about what was happening in my life at this time because I did not want to dwell on the negatives. I needed to maintain a positive mindset, and genuinely believed it would all be well.

My husband dropped me off at the SRH very early on the morning of 15th December. I went to ward D47 and sat in the waiting area, not knowing what to expect. I sat there until one of the ladies came, took me to the ward and showed me my bed. I noticed that they whisked one lady into the surgery theatre, and after that they came for me. I had the re-excision of the margins as well as the sentinel node biopsy, which entailed the removal of the lymph node under my armpit. The sentinel lymph node is the first node in a group of nodes in the body where cancer cells may move to, after they have left the original cancer site. The doctor injects a blue dye or special tracer substance into the area around the original

34

cancer site. The dye or tracer moves to the first lymph node that drains close to the cancer site. The dye makes a map showing areas where the cancer is likely to spread and which lymph node is most likely to have cancer cells. Thus I had two surgeries at the same time, one the sentinel node biopsy and the other, re-excision of margins or wider local excision.

For me, the thought of having 're-excision of margins' was daunting, and the experience was much different from the first one. Given that I had two operations in one go, I was very unwell. When I was taken back to the ward, my eyes were opened to see what women like me were going through. I was in the ward with women whose conditions appeared worse than mine. One of them actually had a mastectomy; another had tubes all over her as her blood was being drained. The most heart-breaking for me was the young lady on the opposite side of my bed who groaned in pain all through the night. Her jaw had been damaged when a tube was being passed through her throat and she was in indescribable pain. I knew I was in the ward for a purpose, but at that point in time, all I needed was sleep. I was feeling very dizzy, slightly faint, and I could hardly open my eyes. Even when my husband and a friend, who was a Consultant at the hospital, visited me at the ward, I barely knew what was happening around me.

My surgery had taken place in the morning. By the time I was taken to the ward, it was nearing visiting hours, at 2.00pm. The lady next to me had lots of people visiting her, so my attempts at sleep were futile. After the visitors left at 5pm, it was time for supper, and shortly after that it would be the next visiting time. I was feeling very exhausted. After visiting time for the day was over, I heaved a sigh of relief and thought I could eventually lie down and have some rest. However, that was wishful thinking. After the visitors left, a couple of the ladies in the ward carried on their conversation. As a light sleeper, I found it difficult to sleep amongst the chatter, but I was so desperately tired, I wanted to cry but was even too weak to do that. I knew I was being kept in the ward so that I could recover fully from the effect of the anesthesia, yet here I was unable to get the sleep I desperately needed. At some point I felt like asking my husband to come and take me home. As a matter of fact, when I was able to manage walking on my own, without support, I went over to the nurses and asked if they had a spare room somewhere where I could sleep. It was approaching 10pm at night, and I had been trying to get some sleep all day. The nurses looked at me as if I was speaking a different language. I think they were rather surprised at my bold request, but sleep deprivation coupled with the operational procedure, can lead to such desperate requests. One of them calmed down and said they would shortly be turning the lights off, and that there were no spare rooms or beds available. They appeared quite hostile. I returned to my ward. As I overheard the conversation between the ladies in the ward, I understood why I had to remain in the ward that night. I told my husband not to bother coming to take me home and that instead when he visited me the next day, he should bring some of my books as I felt it would encourage these women. When I could endure it no longer, I told the ladies that I had been trying to get some sleep all day without much success. I was not being anti-social, but I really needed to sleep. I told them that when I got up in the morning we would have the opportunity to have a real chat, because I found the subject of their discussion quite interesting. Thankfully they understood, and spoke quietly so I could sleep undisturbed.

When I eventually fell asleep in the middle of the night, I heard the lady opposite me groaning all through the night. I think her pain was too overwhelming for her. It made my heart ache so badly. I felt quite helpless, as I was too weak and tired to do anything, however I prayed for her on my bed. In the morning my husband came to visit me and brought copies of my books, which I freely distributed to the ladies in the ward. I shared my faith with the two ladies who had been chatting the previous day. I noticed that a young girl aged about 16 or 17 years arrived and occupied the bed next to mine. I did not know what procedure she had been admitted for, but when the lady next to her bed on the other side told me what it was, I felt compassion for her. I also gave her a copy of my book, but I noticed she was not on her bed when I was leaving. That made me sad as I did not have the opportunity to talk with her.

However, I quietly went over to the bed of the young lady opposite me who had groaned all night, and asked if I could pray for her. She consented, and I did. In a way I was grateful for the opportunity I had to share my faith with these ladies, and to hopefully encourage them in their journey.

Chapter Five

HUG in a Bag?

After my discharge from the hospital, a few friends visited us at home. Some brought me food as they knew I was still recovering from my operation. I will be ever grateful for their thoughtfulness and kindness during this period. I went for my post-op assessment on the 20th of December and met the surgeon and the nurse. I was informed that the result of the nymph node removal was not yet available. Also the MDT had not met, so the treatment plan I would require was still unclear.

I had taken little Christmas presents and thank you cards to this appointment for the Consultant Surgeon and the nurse. In return, the nurse handed me a gift bag, which had the inscription 'HUG in a bag.' This created some curiosity in me, and I was keen to see the contents of the bag. When I got home and brought out the items in the bag, I opened my mouth wide in amazement. I could not believe my eyes. The bag was full of all sorts of goodies for women going through breast cancer treatment. There were some leaflets in the gift bag, which explained the idea behind the concept of 'HUG in a Bag.'

HUG stands for **Help** (a useful list of contacts), **Understanding** (from women who have undergone the same experiences) and **Glamour** (a selection of beauty products). I was deeply moved. This for me is what life is about – using your own experiences to make a difference in the lives of others. Instead of moaning and complaining, others see their experience as an opportunity to help others who face similar situations – making the 'load' much lighter for them when they have to go through a similar encounter. They perceive the 'cup' as 'half-full', instead of 'half-empty'. **HUG in a Bag** is a non-profit organisation formed by three women who met, laughed, cried and supported each other during their treatment for breast cancer. Each of the three coped in their own way, but found that sharing their thoughts, anxieties and concerns was extremely helpful. They also gave each other lots of hugs in times of fear, sadness and joy! The aim of these women is to give 'one more hug in the form of a bag containing gifts, information leaflets and discount vouchers to every person diagnosed with breast cancer in Sunderland Royal Hospital.' This is because they know from their own experience that women can feel very alone and vulnerable at this time and they wanted to show their understanding and support.

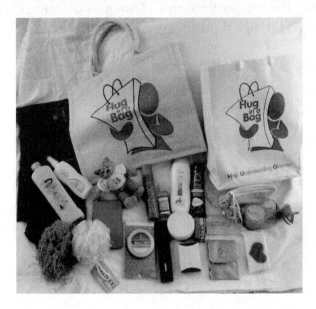

The action of these three women reminds me of a CNN programme (*CNN Heroes*) which my husband and I recently watched. The programme was essentially about people who understood how to turn their trials into triumphs; their pain, into other people's gain. I was particularly touched by the story of the little 12 year old, Jessie Rees, who during her 10 month courageous fight with two brain tumours created 'JOYJARS,' which were used to spread hope, joy and love to children fighting life changing medical illnesses across America in homes and hospitals. She came up with the four-letter word, NEGU, which are now synonymous with the foundation, created after she lost her battle with cancer. NEGU stands for Never Ever Give Up. How inspiring!

This is how we are to treat the trials of life that confront us, to use them as a means for the greater good of man.

When we are facing or have gone through a life changing encounter, our attitude should be 'how can I use this experience to help others? No one should go through what I've been through, and even if they have to go through it, I want to use my experience to help them get through it positively and with dignity.

Chapter Six

Suddenly!

For the past two years, my family had decided that I should have a restful Christmas, and the same happened December 2012. They did not want me cooking and wearing myself out. In addition, some very close friends brought us a very large roast turkey. This was to ensure that I did not have to prepare the turkey either. I was absolutely overwhelmed with the gestures of kindness I received during this period. My younger brother and his family visited us during the Christmas season and we all had a lovely time together. The young lady who prepared the meal did not disappoint at all with her array of dishes for our Christmas meal. She exceeded all expectations.

Generally, my body felt well and strong, and did not show signs of someone recovering from surgery. I still managed to organise Christmas presents for family and friends, although because of the surgery on my breast and on my lymph nodes, I could not drive for some time. However, I was given a leaflet at the hospital showing the regular exercises I needed to do, to ensure I maintained movement in my right arm.

The MDT at SRH still had not met when I went for my next appointment on the 28th of December, according to the Consultant Surgeon who I met with the nurse. However, the stitches on my lymph nodes and alternate stitches on my right breast were removed. I was given another appointment to come to the hospital on the 2nd of January 2013.

On the last Saturday of the year, the 29th of December, I was delighted that I could still take part in the Kids' Club we run in Washington, although I refrained from any vigorous activity. The Kids' Club is one I established that takes place on the last Saturday of the month, in collaboration with a local evangelical church in Washington for children in and around the neighbourhood, in which we engage them in different activities and also taught them stories from the Bible.

I recall that when I was preparing for the second round of surgery, the Consultant had mentioned that one of the risks of the wide local excision was the risk of infection. So, before I went for the surgery, and even on the day itself, my husband and son left no stone unturned when they cleaned the whole house.

We generally celebrate New Year's Eve at church, and use the opportunity to thank God for His protection during the past year. The end of year service on the 31st of December has always been one of my favourites. This particular one was not expected to be an exception. However, on the morning of the 31st of December, as I went into the kitchen to have something to eat, I noticed that my cooking hob needed a bit of cleaning. So I decided to give it a little scrub. As I am right-handed, I cleaned it using my right hand. I thought this small exercise might be of benefit.

After our dinner that evening, I felt quite a bit of pain under my arm and on my right side generally, and was also very tired. My family thought my efforts in cleaning the hob could be what triggered the pain I was experiencing. So I decided that I would take a nap before going to the New Year's Eve service. I chose to lie down on the sofa in our lounge so that I would not sleep past the time we would need to be at the church. However, as I was trying to sleep, I felt very unwell and dizzy, and the pain intensified. I took some painkillers and staggered upstairs and jumped into bed. I told my husband that I would be unable to attend the church service and suggested he could go, and that I would be fine. However, he refused to leave me at home when I was feeling so unwell, so we both stayed home on New Year's Eve.

I woke up on 1 January and felt like I was actually dying. I could not even move myself in bed. That was how bad the pain on my breast was. I could not eat either. I felt feverish and completely helpless. Prior to this time life had been fairly normal despite the various treatments. Not many people knew what I was going through, not even at work or at the Church. Fortunately, the second surgery had taken place close to the Christmas break, so I had no reason to be off sick from work. However, what I was facing at this point in time was different.

I thank God for giving me the strength to get through that day, and much later in the day, I was finally able to wish friends and family a 'Happy New Year'. I went to bed that night, and to my horror the next morning, I discovered that my right breast was dripping with some dirty looking fluid! My clothes were wet as was the bed. I couldn't believe what was happening, and tried to calm the numerous thoughts racing through my mind. Nothing prepared me for this phase in my drama. My right breast was swollen and painfully sore. When the Consultant talked about the risk of infection following the wide local excision, I had no idea what he meant, or what I should expect. Sadly, I did not ask him, either. So, what I encountered on the morning of 2nd January scared the life out of my husband and I.

My husband ran downstairs and brought out some plasters and dressings from our First Aid kit. We put them over the dressing that was there to try to stop the leakage. Fortunately, I had an appointment at the SRH that very day, which was such a welcome relief. We went for the appointment and met the Consultant. A different nurse was there this time as my assigned nurse had mentioned she would be on holiday when I came for my next appointment. The Consultant examined my breast and said there was a build-up of fluid. I was in so much pain as he tried to evacuate the fluid, which was also hot and very messy. He said I had a slight infection, prescribed some antibiotics and a stronger painkiller and I was given some dressing for my wound. For the rest of the week, my husband and I had a routine of waking up in the night to dress my wound, which was always leaking.

I was to examine a PhD thesis in Southampton during the first week of January, and another one at Teeside University in the third week.

I had to email them to have both rescheduled. My next appointment at SRH was scheduled for the 4th of January, and this time my assigned nurse was back. The Consultant tried to squeeze out more pus and to cleanse my breast. The pain I experienced during that period is indescribable. He prescribed a different type of antibiotic. When I asked if I would have to pay again for another prescription, the nurse gave me an NHS Exemption form to fill in so that I would not have to pay for my prescriptions. The fact that I was being offered free medication gave me some concern that my treatment would require a lot of medication. However, I did not see myself as one who would be long-term sick, and as such I did not think I would use the Exemption Certificate for long. Whilst reflecting on the infection in my wound, the nurse said she had not seen one so bad. This would explain the level of pain I encountered!! That was a real experience for me, and one that I will never forget. Again, it appeared that everything about my diagnosis and the outcome were unique, however my faith in God never waivered.

The first Saturday of the month was usually when the Overseas Fellowship of Nigerian Christians (OFNC) had their regular meeting. The OFNC is a national body of mostly (but not exclusively) Nigerian Christians residing in the UK. It is a fellowship that not only provides support for its members, but also actively involved in different community initiatives nationally and internationally. My husband and I were scheduled to lead the first meeting of the year. Unfortunately I was not in a position to attend, so he went without me. The Branch Co-ordinator and another family came to visit after the meeting, bringing me some food, for which I was very grateful.

My next hospital appointment was on the 9th of January. The last few stitches on my breast were removed, and the procedure was quite painful. The Consultant advised that my treatment would be followed up with radiotherapy. He said it was necessary to follow up such procedures with radiotherapy to ensure that the tumour does not return. 'Radio…what?' I thought within myself. I had heard of radiotherapy, chemotherapy and the like, but I never thought it was something I would experience in my life. I felt like saying to the Consultant, 'Oh! Don't worry, I'll be fine; I don't think I'll need that.' But, of course I trusted he knew what he was doing. I trusted God that the treatment would be a success. Before we left, I gave both the Consultant and the nurse a copy each of my book, *The Greatest Debtor to His Love – and a Trophy of His Grace.* I told the nurse that another book would emerge from my experience. She gave me some leaflets to help me understand my radiotherapy treatment and what it would entail.

On Saturday, 12 January 2013, I checked my wound and found it was completely dry. What a relief! I would no longer need to administer the dressing. This meant that I could actually have a real shower without any fear of my wound being wet. Wow!!! What a great feeling!! These are the little things we take for granted.

My younger sister had visited us the previous week and brought me some fruit juices, including beetroot juice. I use beetroot in my salad regularly but had never drunk it in the form of a juice. I took a small glass before I left for work on Friday, 18th of January. That evening, I was still at work, and after visiting the toilet, I was petrified by what I saw in that bowl. I know I have had near death encounters and experiences that made the BBC Reporter describe my life as 'dramatic and eventful.' The discharge from my breast did scare me, but I don't think that compared with how I felt on this particular evening. When you're undergoing treatment for what is described as a 'rare form of cancer,' anything can happen. In fact, you don't know what to expect anymore. The liquid in the toilet bowl was pure red! I feared the worst. I could not remove my stare at the toilet bowl. I told myself that there was no way I would not get these specimens tested. I called up my husband who was doing some work in the library at the time. I told him what had happened and that I needed to go the Accident and Emergency immediately so they could test my urine. Again I felt like death was probably around the corner, and that some of the organs in my body had been badly damaged and that I was bleeding internally. Oh! The feeling was horrible!

I cannot recall how many times and for how long I stared into the toilet bowl. However, as I was walking back to my room, I felt the urge within me to phone my younger sister to ask her a few questions. I asked her if she was aware of the effect from drinking beetroot juice? I told her what had just happened to me. She said she was sorry she had not alerted me as to what I should expect after drinking beetroot juice; that your urine will be coloured red, like blood. My Goodness! What a huge relief! I rang my husband and told him not to panic as I had confirmed with my sister the reason for the change in my urine. That experience was overwhelming, and I would not wish for anyone to feel the way I felt that evening.

My last appointment at the SRH before the commencement of my radiotherapy treatment was on the 23rd of January. After examining me, the Consultant said I would be receiving a letter from the Freemans Hospital in Newcastle giving details of my radiotherapy treatment. I would also be receiving a letter from them inviting me for a review of my progress after six months.

Chapter Seven

This is Reality

On the 24th of January, I received a phone call from a member of staff at Freemans Hospital to schedule an appointment for my radiotherapy. An appointment was fixed for the 31st of January.

I thought I had enough trouble already with all the challenges I had faced in the past few months, so when another terrible pain developed on the left side of my neck close to my throat on Monday, 28th January after my marathon teaching session, I was very upset. I couldn't understand where the pain had come from. Initially I thought the pain was on my gum and I used Bonjela for two days. I placed my hands on my neck and prayed. I also took some painkillers. I felt some relief, but as I was teaching on Wednesday, 30th of January, the pain was unbearable. I called my dentist to make an appointment thinking it was something to do with my gum. However the time scheduled for the appointment (2.10pm) coincided with the time (2.00pm) I had scheduled to see my PhD students. I was not happy with that arrangement. On second thoughts, I called my GP's surgery for an emergency appointment. They offered me one at 1.10pm. I thought that was a much better timing and then cancelled the appointment with the dentist. I told them I needed to see my GP first and that if he felt it was a dental problem, then I would come back to him.

I went for my appointment with my GP and we both looked at each other. I could feel tears trickling down my cheeks. We both remembered the last time I was there with all that had transpired since that first meeting and the confirmation of the lump in my breast on Friday, 12th October. I had not been back to his surgery since then. He always used the expression 'it is well!' Of course I understood what he meant. He had been inundated with letters from the Consultant looking after me at SRH giving him updates on my treatment since the discovery of the lump in my breast. As my GP, it was important for him to be kept up to date with the treatment I was receiving and the different outcomes.

Since most of my classroom teaching was in the second semester, my radiotherapy treatment would affect some of my classes. Prior to this time only my Associate Dean knew I had gone in for surgery a couple of times. In spite of this, I was still in and out of work as much as possible. It so happened that the worst part of my illness took place during the Christmas break when the University was on holiday. This meant that none of my colleagues at work knew I was undergoing treatment for cancer. I was back at work in January like everyone else when the University resumed. Given that one of my teaching sessions would be affected during my treatment, I had to alert the Associate Dean, the Resources Manager and my Team Leader so they could make arrangements for someone to cover some of my classes.

I recall how shocked my Team Leader was when I told him I was going for post-op treatment at the Freeman Hospital. He said he was unaware that I had undergone surgery. Again, no one asked what type of treatment I was going for, so there was no need to disclose this. I thank God for this. I know that some members of my family and even some friends had asked why I did not consider taking time off work given what was happening in my life. I know some ladies who had given up work for six months after receiving the type of diagnosis that I had. I recall telling someone that I believed God was going to heal me, and I didn't want to sit at home when I could be living my life.

On Thursday, 31 January I went for 'Treatment Planning', which I had heard so much about. Our eldest son was off work that day so he drove me to the hospital as my husband had work commitments. I had been reading about radiotherapy to familiarise myself with what to expect, therefore when the Consultant Oncologist at the Newcastle Centre for Cancer Care (NCCC) explained the procedure, it sounded familiar to me. What was interesting was the comment the Consultant made when she was looking through my notes. She said 'this is the lady whose story has gone all over the country.' She said that even the National Pathologist put an exclamation mark in her comments, as she had never encountered the type of lump that was removed from my breast before.

Sometimes we can be so distant from what goes on in the lives of others until it gets close to home. How often had I received leaflets through our letterbox to support Macmillan Cancer Trust, or Marie Curie Cancer Care, or other charities aimed at people suffering from cancer? Did I understand the magnitude of the impact of cancer on the lives of others, until I visited this Centre? Not really. How many precious lives do you know that have been cut short through cancer? It is not easy for anyone to understand the impact that cancer has in the lives of people until it gets close to you. I recall that as we drove into the Freeman Hospital, I didn't know what to expect. I didn't even know that such a place (the NCCC) existed, that specially catered for people under going cancer treatment. It is well worth visiting that place, as it drives reality home. The experience was quite humbling.

My first radiotherapy treatment was on Tuesday 26th of February. The hospital had tried to arrange my treatment around my husband's work schedule as well as those of others who would be giving me daily lifts to the hospital (Monday to Friday) for three weeks. I was told that one of the side effects of radiotherapy was fatigue. The suggestion was that I should stay off work for three weeks during my treatment. In preparation for my treatment, I set aside some time to pray. I prayed that the radiotherapy treatment would not harm my body in any way; neither would I suffer any side effects from it. I believe God heard my prayer.

I had different people taking me for my daily treatment; my husband, eldest son, second son, and a friend. The sheer number of people who attend treatment for one form of cancer or another in that place is staggering. I was pleased that two of our sons had the experience of visiting NCCC, so that they would understand what was going on in the lives of others around us. One intriguing aspect of it all was that these people receiving radiotherapy just looked like ordinary people that we would walk past on the street and not look twice. How many people in my place of work had any idea of what was going on in my life? Not one!

This reminds me of the day I had my first surgery on the 20th of November 2012. As I sat in the hospital lounge at the SRH waiting for my husband to come and collect me after my first operation, I picked up one of the magazines ('*Heart Matters*') on the table that had caught my attention. One of the features in the magazine was the experience of a 68-year-old lady who wrote about how she was still trying to make the most of her life in spite of her personal circumstances - she had suffered two heart attacks, undergone a divorce, and although still close to her ex-husband, he had died. Worse still, she had lost her only son, a 24-year-old deep-sea diver, who had failed to return from one of his diving expeditions. As a mother of three sons myself, I could not imagine what that must feel like. Usually when you lose a loved one, you can put closure to it by giving them a befitting burial, but what happens when every day you wake up trying to imagine what must have befallen your most loved, and only child?

As I was thinking about this, my mind also went to the BBC Panorama programme (I think it was called 'Mind Reader'), which featured some families who were faced with the challenges of caring for their sons who had been involved in accidents causing brain damage. It was difficult for me to try to imagine what such a challenge must feel like. It was so humbling to watch these families love and care for their loved-one so deeply, despite the difficulty they faced.

As we drove home from hospital, I said to my husband, "we have no idea what people are going through!," I told him about what I had read in the magazine and recalled the BBC Panorama programme as well. In my own case, here I was coming out of hospital following surgery, after having been in and out of hospital for some 4-5 weeks undergoing all sorts of tests and finding the prospect of surgery rather daunting. Yet I went about my duties as normal, putting the needs of others before mine, and trying to do all I could to get on with life in spite of what was happening. Not many knew I was facing such a health challenge in my own life. I also knew there were things I wish I could do that I was unable to.

The fact is that every single person we come across is facing a challenge. It could be physical, mental, emotional, financial or otherwise. This is why we must be careful about jumping to conclusions about people. We must never judge or condemn others because we have no clue what is going on in their lives. We all need to have a more caring attitude and to be nice to people - a kind word, a smile, etc. We cannot underestimate the impact of such seemingly small gestures. Rather than judge wrongly, criticise or condemn others, let us whisper a prayer for them and ask God to help them in whatever issue they face, because we do not know the issues they are dealing with.

How can I forget a personal experience a few years back when I met a homeless middle-aged man who had stumbled into an event gathering looking for help and no one took any notice of him? I went gently to him and placed my hands on his shoulders. This man looked straight into my eyes and asked "Is there hope for someone like me?" My, oh my! Can I ever forget how much I wept that day and how this man wept also? After I calmed down, I held him closely and told him there was hope for him, and I shared God's love with him. To cut the story short, this man (John) prayed and made the decision to trust God with his life. After this, he appeared more calm and peaceful, and the immediate transformation of his countenance was visible for all to see. We gave him a Bible and continued to support him, where possible.

We can use the trials and challenges we face in life to help others. No one is immune from trouble. The issue is how we react to our challenges and difficulties.

Chapter Eight

Know Who You Are

The importance of knowing who you really are is an essential part of your everyday interactions with people. If you were walking down a street and someone tried to get your attention by shouting 'Mary', when your name is Lucy, would you turn? Perhaps not! In the same way, when one is facing a cancer challenge, knowing who you really are will play an important part in managing the whole process. One of the factors that enabled me to stand up to cancer was the fact that I knew who I was. It was Dr Phil Mcgraw who said 'unless you know who you are, you will always be vulnerable to what people say'. This is particularly relevant when a person has been diagnosed with cancer.

I know a few people who when they were diagnosed with cancer, the wall around them literally collapsed. Their lives came to a stop more or less. This should not be if you truly know who you are. From the moment I found the lump in breast, I had no doubt in mind about who I was, a winner, and a survivor! Whether or not I was told that the lump found in my breast was malignant cancer, it didn't matter at all. I wasn't going to be overtaken by fear because I knew who I was, and that God was with me. This was why I didn't think it was necessary to discuss my diagnosis with many people, as I was confident that all would be well.

One of the advantages of being a person of faith is that your life and everything about you is built around your faith or belief. As a Christian, I believe in God, and in what the Bible says about me. There are many bible passages that have promises that help one cope with different challenges that we face in life. For example, in John 1:12, the Bible says *'But as many as received Him, to them He gave the right to become children of God, to those who believe in His name'*. This tells me that if I know who I am - a child of God, then I expect my Father to protect me, like every earthly father would protect his child. Therefore, whether or not I was facing a life-threatening disease, I knew I was under the protection of my Father God.

It is possible that there are many out there, who do not believe in God, or in the Bible, and yet know who they are, and face their cancer challenge differently; that is perfectly okay. I am simply sharing what helped me through one of the most difficult periods in my life. As a matter of fact, the following promises in the Bible come to mind: *"who shall separate us from the love of Christ? Shall tribulation, or distress, or persecution, or famine, or nakedness, or peril, or sword? ...Yet in all these things we are more than conquerors through Him who loved us. For I am persuaded that neither death nor life, nor angels nor principalities nor powers, nor things present nor things to come, nor height nor depth, nor any other created thing, shall be able to separate us from the love of God...* (Romans 8: 35-39). How can one have such words of reassurance and harbor fear?

Another incredible promise is found in Isaiah 43:1-4, which says *"Fear not, for I have redeemed you; I have called you by your name; You are Mine. When you pass through the waters, I will be with you; and through the rivers, they shall not overflow you. When you walk through the fire, you shall not be burned, nor shall the flame scorch you. For I am the Lord your God,... since you were precious in My sight, you have been honoured, and I have loved you...".* Wow!!! How can anyone have such words of comfort and reassurance and fear what the doctors say?

Knowing that I am loved, that I am a child of God, helped me a lot. As a matter of fact, the story of my life from my mother's womb has been extra-ordinary. So when I was diagnosed with malignant, life-threatening cancer, I knew God was with me. Besides, knowing how many times He had delivered me from near-death encounters was a great encouragement. I wasn't prepared to allow cancer to define my life. As Oprah Winfrey rightly said 'don't be confused between what people say you are and who you know you are'. I had no doubt in mind, who I was.

If you ever have the misfortune of being diagnosed with cancer, it is important that you know who you are, and that you do not allow the cancer to define you. We can all stand up to cancer if we truly know who we are.

Chapter Nine

The Power of the Mind

Statistics has it that one in three people will suffer from cancer at one time or other in their life time. If anyone had told me that I would ever have breast cancer, I would never have believed it, more so, since no female in my family line has ever suffered from cancer. So why do some people suffer from cancer and others don't? It is a question which has no simple answer.

Cancer is a complex group of diseases with many possible causes, some of which are hereditary, whilst others are associated with individual lifestyle factors. Even if one cannot avoid cancers that are genetic, we can all do something about making changes to our lifestyles to avoid those cancers which are avoidable.

So what happens if after you've taken all precautions you still end up unexpectedly being diagnosed with cancer? Does your life suddenly come to a standstill, or to an end? I still recall the shock I had when I discovered the lump in my breast. And it's not just me; everyone who is diagnosed with cancer experiences that same shock. Cancer is the 'C' word that no one wants to be associated with. The sad thing also about cancer is that for some people, by the time they discover they have it, it's almost too late; it has spread to other organs in the body, and the person is given a limited time to live.

However, what happens to us from the moment we receive the 'news' will most often than not determine the outcome, and this is where our mind is key. I know people who were diagnosed with terminal cancer who are still alive today because of the power of their mind. There is no underestimating what our human mind can accomplish. It was James Allen who said, *"You are today where your thoughts have brought you; you will be tomorrow where your thoughts take you,"*

Scientists have proved that we can use our brain to improve the quality of our lives, and we can lower our stress levels by managing our thoughts. Your thoughts are powerful and they frame the triumphs or tragedies of your life. We can also heal ourselves through positive thinking. In the Bible, it says 'for as a man thinks in his heart, so is he…' (Proverbs 23:7)

This means that when we have the right attitude and think positively, we can manage and win the battle over cancer. In fact, high stress levels and negative (toxic) thoughts are like poison that can cause cancer.

In my own case, as soon as I received the diagnosis of breast cancer, I knew I wasn't going to accept it; neither was I going to let it affect the quality of my life. It is not usual that someone is diagnosed with cancer and her work colleagues or even close friends and associates are not aware of it. To make matters worse, the kind of cancer that I was diagnosed with was described as "very very rare". An extract of one of the letters sent to my GP, dated 19/12/2012 read:

Dear Dr …

"I reviewed this lady in the follow up breast clinic today. She had her excision of right breast lump on 20th November 2012. Histology wise she has got a lump which is very very rare variety of mucinous adenocarcinoma and this is ER/PR negative. I have discussed it with Dr…, Consultant Histopathologist in Sunderland Royal Hospital. She did send the specimen to Dr… in Queen Elizabeth Hospital and she commented she has not seen anything like that before but she pointed out there is a possibility there might be a primary tumour on ovary appendix and pancreas. Dr … pointed out that we should go ahead and do a CT scan of the abdomen, thorax and pelvis. This specimen has been sent to Dr … the Consultant

Histopathologist, the National expert in London for reconfirmation...."

The picture painted in this correspondence is enough to cause anyone to panic, and to fear the worst. As if that was not bad enough, I received the following letter from a surgical trainee at Sunderland Royal Hospital, dated 14/11/12, which read:

"Dear Mrs Okike
I am one of the surgical trainees at Sunderland Royal Hospital working for Mr... and the Breast Surgery team. I am writing to you regarding your recent breast surgery. The nature of the lump that was removed is very rare and I would like your permission to write up the case for submission to a medical journal for publication. Please find enclosed a copy of the proposed case report for submission as well as two copies of the consent form...

In addition to the enclosed text, there may well be some images of the pathology slides included in the final report; these will be fully anonymised also. Please note some changes may be made to the text; these will not compromise your anonymity.

Many thanks again for your kind help with this. If you have any questions please contact me.

Yours sincerely
....

Further, the case report noted that "Primary Mammary Mucinous Cystadenocarcinoma is a very rare, recently described condition with few cases in the literature and a small body of evidence upon which to base treatment decisions".

How many people are diagnosed with cancer and have their case published in the British Medical Journal? These evidences suggest that from every perspective, the diagnosis I had received had the potential to cause fear and anxiety, in addition to the cancer itself. Nevertheless, I kept a positive attitude, which was very important.

In fact, my MDT managing my case were often surprised and regularly commented that I was really coping well.

My faith in God provided me with the positive attitude necessary to enable me to stand up to the cancer challenge.

When I was undergoing my treatment, I went about business as normal. Sometimes I went for my radiotherapy treatment from work, and at other times I would go for my treatment and then go to work from there.

No soldier goes into battle with defeat on his/her mind. A positive attitude is key to winning all of life's battles and challenges.

Chapter Ten

The Power of Words

Besides our thoughts, our words also shape the outcome of our lives, and there is a connection between our thoughts and our words. In the Bible it says '...*what you say flows from what is in your heart.* (Luke 6:45) (NLT)*,* which means that the words you speak are a reflection of your thoughts. Both your thoughts and your words have the power to influence your life, therefore, if we expect good outcomes, we must speak the right words. For example, even if you went to the doctor and received a negative report about your health, you have a choice over what you believe, how you choose to respond, and the type of people you invite to accompany you on this journey. The Bible says "*death and life are in the power of the tongue, and those who love it will eat its fruits'* (Proverbs 18:21). '*Those who guard their lips preserve their lives, but those who speak rashly will come to ruin.'* (Proverbs 13:3)

These passages in the Bible make it clear that your words are the vehicles with which you express and share your experiences with others, and they inevitably affect your experience. This is why when I was diagnosed with breast cancer; I chose not to tell many people. I was not even prepared to talk about it, or mention the word cancer in my conversation because I knew I had already won the battle in my mind. The only way my colleagues or those outside of my immediate family circle will ever find out that I was ever diagnosed with cancer and went through cancer treatment is when they read this book. I did not want to give cancer power over me.

I've often been shocked when I've heard people say things like 'The doctor says I've only got few months to live,' and they resolve themselves to that fact. A positive response to such a report would be the Bible passage that states '*I shall not die but live, and declare the works of the Lord...*' (Psalm 118:17). Another helpful response could be '*with long life You will satisfy me and show me Your salvation'* (Psalm 91:16). The fact is that you don't need to be a person of any faith to use these words. If you believe that your words will influence your life, you can search for positive words to speak over your situation. There are many books out there on the power of positive thinking that can help you develop a positive mindset.

I used the Bible as my reference point because of my faith, and because I see it as God's words of reassurance to me, in every situation. It is 'a lamp to my feet, and a light that lightens my path' (Psalm 119: 105), which means it guides me, and gives me hope.

Have you heard the story of David and Goliath? It is about a young man, David, who killed a mighty giant, named Goliath. The Israelites were engaged in battle with the Philistines, and the latter, had Goliath on their side, who intimidated and threatened the Israelites daily. David was the youngest son of Jesse, and he had been sent on an errand by his father, to go and inquire about the welfare of his three brothers, who were engaged in battle on the side of the Israelites. It was whilst on this errand that he overheard the threat of Goliath, challenging the Israelites to present a man, who would take him on in battle, and whoever defeated the other, brought victory to the rest of army. Whereas the Israelites were all scared to death by the size and the threat of Goliath, the Philistine, the little lad, David, would not be intimidated by his threats. He first defeated the giant in his mind and with his words before he threw his sling (1Samuel 17). His string, which he threw in the name of his God, brought the giant tumbling down, and victory to the Israelites.

Given the very rare nature of the cancer with which I was diagnosed, it would have been very easy for me to be downcast and seek sympathy from many friends, however, I chose to believe the words of life and hope from the Bible. I was ready to stand up to cancer, and I did. Faith in God and in the assurance of His love for me was all I needed.

Anyone can stand up to cancer. You simply need to cultivate the habit of thinking positively and saying the right words. The glass can be half full or half empty; it depends on which perspective you choose to adopt. Therefore, you need to exercise yourself in the practice of renewing your mind and the words that you speak daily. If you speak defeat, you will experience defeat. If you speak life, you will receive life.

Chapter Eleven

You are What You Do and Eat

There are different types of cancer, and they all have one thing in common – they are caused by uncontrolled growth of the cells in our bodies. Research suggests that cancer can be hereditary or can originate from lifestyle factors. Whilst much progress has been made through medical science and technology in addressing the threat of cancer and in searching for a lasting cure for the disease, there are steps we can all take to reduce the risk of getting cancer, including changing our lifestyle.

Another way that I stood up to cancer after my diagnosis was to re-examine my habits and lifestyle, especially since there was no history of breast cancer in my family line. I made necessary adjustments to my diet and tried to increase my level of physical activity, such as taking the stairs rather than lifts at work and elsewhere, whenever possible. I also examined my life to see if there were any stress-related activities that I was engaged in that could have triggered the disease, and gave them up.

Cancer can be beaten, if it is diagnosed early. This means we all need to pay more attention to our bodies and look out for symptoms, such as unexplained or persistent changes. This includes unusual lumps or swelling, unexplained weight loss, breathlessness or blood in the urine or bowels. Whilst these are not the only symptoms, spotting cancer early is important as it means treatment is more likely to be successful. Therefore it is important to seek medical advice as soon as you notice any unusual symptoms in your body. If the cancer has spread, treatment becomes more difficult, and generally a person's chances of surviving are much lower. This was why I was desperate to make an appointment with my GP once I felt the lump in my breast that fateful day. Although anyone can develop cancer, it is more common as we get older. Usually 9 out of 10 cases are in people aged 50 or over.

Experts estimate that more than 4 in 10 cancer cases could be prevented by lifestyle changes. Once you have the misfortune of being diagnosed with cancer, you pay closer attention to what you do and eat. Cancer diagnosis usually calls for self-examination, and life-style adjustments. But why wait until you're diagnosed with cancer to start addressing your life-style and diet? Just as you are what you think and say, you are also what you do and eat. Avoiding cancer or undergoing treatment for cancer also calls for self-discipline in what we do and eat. We have heard it from various quarters that bad habits such as smoking or excessive alcohol consumption increases our risk of cancer. Also, eating the wrong types of food increases cancer risk.

Research provides evidence that inadequate exercise or physical activity can increase your weight, which can affect hormone levels and your immunity system. When you pay close attention to your health, you are playing your part in minimising the risk of cancer.

I'm not a health expert, but I know how much effort I've made in trying to keep fit, and eating the right things. There is a lot of information online about what to eat and what not to eat in order to avoid the risk of cancer. It is advisable that you educate yourself on the causes of different types of cancer, take reasonable steps, and make adjustments in your lifestyle to avoid them as much as possible.

In our home for example, we do not eat fried foods; we roast and grill instead. Also, we do not consume or serve alcohol. We take plenty of fruits and vegetables and avoid fatty foods. It's only occasionally that I serve red meat such as lamb, and we avoid processed foods as much as possible. I make my own fruit juices and don't consume fizzy drinks or foods with high sugar content.

You can stand up to cancer by watching your lifestyle and diet. Whilst living a healthy lifestyle isn't a guarantee against cancer, nevertheless, it helps to stack the odds in your favour. Don't wait until you're diagnosed with cancer to stand up to it. Prevention is better than cure.

ABOUT THE AUTHOR

Dr Elewechi Ngozi Okike is an inspirational writer, who works within the higher education sector. She has been in academia for over 35 years, and is passionate about making a difference to the lives of others. This is reflected in all her writings.

Her desire to make a difference in the lives of others led to the establishment of BOOK AID FOR AFRICA, a Charity that is helping to address the imbalance in educational provision in Africa.

www.bookaidforafrica.com

BUY ONLINE AT
www.assurancepublications.com
www.amazon.com
ORDER BY PHONE
0191 4167883 or 07799653641

Visit www.assurancepublications.com to read an interview with Dr. Ngozi Okike, exclusive extracts and many more

ALSO BY THE AUTHOR

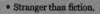

The Greatest Debtor to His Love

and a Trophy of His Grace

- Stranger than fiction.
- Real and captivating!
- Highly inspirational and challenging.
- Unlocks secrets for overcoming obstacles and challenges
- Contains keys for WINNING in life.
- Sarah Hathaway of BBC Tyne describes Ngozi's life as 'very dramatic and eventful',

How does anyone survive abortion, escape rape, murder, abduction and overcome prejudice and injustice? Find out as you read this real life account of Elewechi Ngozi Okike in "The Greatest Debtor to His Love and a Trophy of His Grace".

This is a book that encourages one never to give up on one's dreams and aspirations, even in the face of persecution, no matter how long it takes. It is a compelling read, both in style and content.

ALSO BY THE AUTHOR

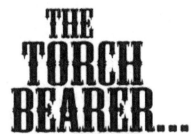

TWO SIDES OF THE STORY

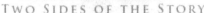

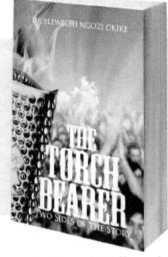

- A captivating read!
- Highly inspirational
- Recognizing your 'God moment'
- Avoid presumptuousness
- There's nothing wrong with recognition
- Faith accomplishes the impossible
- Shine your light even in the darkest moments
- See beyond the veil; appearances are deceptive

Elewechi Ngozi Okike rejected an opportunity to be one of the Torch Bearers to carry the Olympic Torch, as part of the opening of the London 2012 Olympics. While she was musing over this decision, she suddenly found herself facing a breast cancer diagnosis. So, how do you shine your light and carry your torch for all to see in the face of a life-threatening disease?

Through the experiences shared in the book, Elewechi helps the reader to appreciate the importance and the significance of being 'Torch Bearers' even in the most difficult and dark places in life. She draws attention to the fact that our ability to shine our light at such times has a higher level impact than carrying the physical Olympic Torch.

ALSO BY THE AUTHOR

Your New Life
A HANDY GUIDE TO SUCCESSFUL CHRISTIAN LIVING

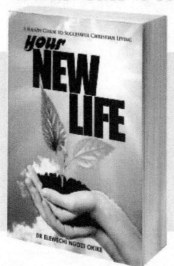

- A manual for effective discipleship
- Invaluable for mature and new believers
- A handy guide for successful Christian living
- Effective for making people true followers of Jesus Christ
- Written in easy to understand language
- Helps new believers go on to maturity
- A must have manual for every Church or Christian organization with a passion for souls

This manual is a vital tool for those who desire to fulfill the commission of Jesus Christ to 'Make disciples and teach them to obey my commands'. It is also a handy guide for new believers who desire to live a successful Christian life. God is not just interested in seeing souls get saved, He is also interested in seeing them established in their faith.

This book is for every church, organisation or individual, passionate about seeing souls saved and nurtured in the faith. It is a book not just for new believers, but for every Christian desiring a strong foundation in their walk with God and a fruitful Christian life.

Made in the
USA
Monee, IL